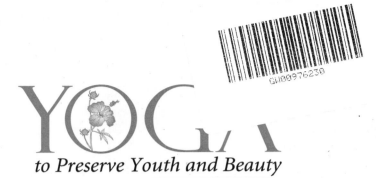

YOGA

to Preserve Youth and Beauty

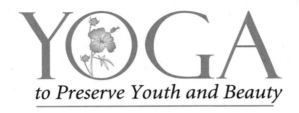

YOGA
to Preserve Youth and Beauty

BIJOYLAXMI HOTA

Rupa & Co

Text Copyright © Bijoylaxmi Hota 2004
Copyright © Rupa & Co. 2004

First Published 2004
Second Impression 2005

Published by

Rupa & Co

7/16 Ansari Road, Daryaganj
New Delhi 110 002

Sales Centres
Allahabad, Bangalore, Chandigarh, Chennai,
Hyderabad, Jaipur, Kathmandu,
Kolkata, Mumbai, Pune

ISBN: 81-291-0266-8

Printed in India by
Gopsons Papers Ltd.
A-14 Sector 60
Noida 201 301

Thanks to
Swami Swaroopananda Saraswati Bhubaneswar
Dr. P. K. Misra (Ram Manohar Lohia Hospital, New Delhi)-for verifying the
contents of the book.

Photography
Sanjay Taneja (cover)

Models
Reela Hota (Odissi Danseuse)
Divyanshu Sharma

Make-up
Meenakshi Dutt

Designed and illustrated by
Ishtihaar, New Delhi

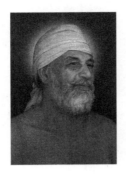

With the blessings
of my Guru and Guide

Paramahamsa Swami Satyananda Saraswati

Contents

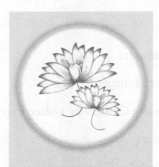

Introduction

INTRODUCTION

I remember the first time I saw my guru Paramahamsa Swami Sri Satyananda Saraswati. He was giving a spiritual discourse in my home town. What struck me first about him was his amazing appearance. Even at sixty, his body was so muscular and so well toned! His skin was literally glowing; and it seemed incredibly smooth, like a baby's. He was so impressive and handsome that my ten-year-old daughter lost her heart to him. And, when I wanted to leave after the discourse was over, she wouldn't budge! She was ready to follow him to the end of the world.

The exterior is but the reflection of the various aspects of the interior—a fact which mankind has never fully appreciated. Since antiquity they have chased the dream to be beautiful and to remain youthful forever. They have tried every conceivable means to fulfil their wish. If Cleopatra bathed in milk and Noorjehan in rose water; today's generation is injecting neuro-toxins into the body, snipping away portions of the skin and sucking out kilos of fat. Adipose tissues have become the source of anxiety and stress all over the world. A fortune is spent by thousands of people on beauty products like lotions and potions which focus only on the exterior.

The cause of a beauty problem may lie at any level in the

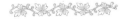

multilevelled personality of a human being. Dark circles around the eyes could be due to constipation or lack of sleep; hair loss could be because of tension or hormonal imbalance; an emotional problem may lead to compulsive eating disorder resulting in weight gain; and a psychological problem may erupt out as rashes. In such cases, external treatment may help temporarily but cannot be a permanent cure. Only when the root cause of the problem is removed, does it naturally disappear. And yoga is one of the systems that has the means to deal with each level of personality effectively.

To mention a few cases—a young grossly overweight girl, who was not losing even an ounce, in spite of an extremely low-calorie diet came to me for treatment. I taught her a relaxation technique and made her do *Guru Shankha Prakshyalan* – a cleansing *kriya*. She lost twelve kilos in fifteen days and has stayed that way since.

Another case is that of a Czech lady who too had an overweight problem, but for a different reason. She was munching the whole day long. No matter how much she tried to curb her urge for food, she was not able to do so. I told her to make a resolution during yogic relaxation and not to eat out of turn. After 10-15 days I overheard her advising her friend in the class to practise the same method of losing weight. She proudly announced that with the resolution during yogic relaxation she had overcome her own problem. Let me also mention the flip side of this story. Despite my instructing her to use only positive words for her resolve, she had framed a negative sentence — 'I will not eat so much'. The result was — whenever she thought of food, she got cramps in her stomach! Luckily, I overheard that too, and told her how to rectify it.

The third case that comes to my mind is that of a growing girl with hair all over her body. I concentrated on her glandular system, and taught her the relevant *asanas, pranayama* and meditation. I also advised her to talk to her body after meditation (technique described in the last chapter). When I saw her after a few years it was quite apparent that it had worked!

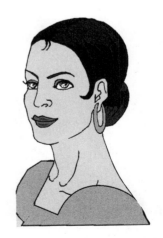

But, yoga was never devised to beautify the body. All that it aims is to maintain perfect health to help the practitioner progress in his or her spiritual path with ease. In the process it normalises the glandular functions, purifies the blood, trims the body, tones up the system, increases energy or *prana*, relaxes the mind, clears the psyche and drives away negativity. The result is a supple body, good health and the radiance of a good person.

As degeneration sets in with ill health it is easily

arrested with perfect physical, mental and psychological health. At the same time, certain yogic techniques promote tissue regeneration. And thus the ageing process of the body is considerably slowed down.

Yoga's effectiveness in preserving tissue health is so great that it can even stretch beyond the physical death of a person as was seen in the case of the great Yogi Paramahamsa Sri Yogananda. The Yogi took *mahasamadhi*, or willed demise, on the March 7, 1952 in Los Angeles. His body was kept under observation in a local mortuary.

To the profound astonishment of all, the body did not decay at all. It remained fresh and odourless even after twenty days, when his coffin was finally closed.

Achieving such a feat as that of the Paramahamsa may or may not be possible for an ordinary person but, yoga, proper diet and observation of certain health rules go a long way in preserving the practitioner's health, youth and beauty for a long time. Most yoga practitioners bear the proof of this.

Yoga is a vast system with various techniques which besides being confusing, make it impossible to practise them all everyday. This book, *Yoga to Preserve Youth and Beauty* will help you identify your problem areas and choose the relevant yogic techniques. Also included are some traditional rituals and practices of ancient India which too contribute to good health and beauty. Frame your own routine and follow it with sincerity – the result will be for you to see.

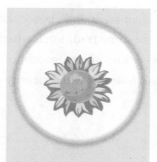

Trimmers

CHAPTER I

Extremely high calorie diet and lack of adequate physical activities have led to one of the major problems of the developed countries — obesity. Obese parents transmit their genes to their offsprings, making them obese as well. These children with too many fat cells in the body, rarely lose weight, exposing themselves to various problems in life.

First, obesity puts excessive strain on the system as each gland and organ has to work much more than it is designed to. The heart has to work overtime to supply blood to these glands and organs for their extra work. At the same time, the extra fat cells and muscle cells too need blood for them which again the heart has to provide. Making the heart work so much can lead to its exhaustion which could prove fatal.

Secondly, mental and psychological problems may also manifest in overweight people. Their features look heavy and unattractive, making them look older. This often causes a lack of self-esteem in them, which in turn can lead to other behavioural problems. They may shun people; care less about their appearance and health and get into a depression.

On the other hand, a trim and well-proportioned

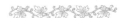

body is a great asset. It promotes good health; it is pleasing to the eyes; and it is a moral booster. It draws the admiration of every beholder, whether or not its owner is bestowed with classical beauty features. All this helps the person acquire better self-confidence and sail through life with ease.

To combat obesity, taking a low calorie diet is the first step. Most of the modern slimming diets which are being marketed worldwide emphasise on certain constituents at the cost of some others, which can cause serious health problems. Some recommend eliminating carbohydrates from the diet altogether and concentrate on proteins. A protein rich diet increases uric acid in the body as the end product of all proteins is uric acid. Too much of this acid can put tremendous burden on the kidneys and damage them. It can also lead to ailments such as arthritis and gout.

Excluding carbohydrates from the diet has its own problems. Carbohydrates are the chief source of energy for body tissues. If this food is excluded, all the tissues including those of the brain are starved, which is undesirable. Excluding fat from diet too is harmful. It hampers the absorption of fat-soluble vitamins. Also, body hormones are made from fat. In its absence their secretion is inadequate. As all the activities of the system are regulated by

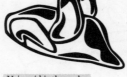

Uric acid is the end
product of proteins

hormones, their insufficiency can cause various problems. Hence, having a balanced diet is essential for good health.

Therefore, have your own dietary chart. Avoid high-calorie food such as refined flour, refined sugar, fried food and excess fat.

Adequate physical exercise is equally important to trim the body. Normal exercise, if overdone, can cause more harm than good. Whereas there is no danger of overdoing yogic exercises. In fact yogic exercises make the body stronger while trimming it down. Hence it is wiser to play safe and practise yoga, which has been around for centuries proving its worth.

The following yogasanas are dynamic in nature which affect all parts of the body equally effectively.

Surya Namaskar

This is one of the most effective yogic exercise, which stretches, massages and trims down the body in the shortest possible time. Unlike other asanas Surya Namaskar can be practised as many as 108 rounds, though 20-50 rounds are more common. The best thing about Surya Namaskar is that one does not lose energy practising this exercise so many times; rather one gains it, i.e. the more you do it the more energetic you feel.

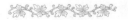

I once suggested it to a girl whose energy level was not too high, though, being a classical dancer she needed extra energy for her daily practise. Every day after her dance session, she would just flop into bed listless. When I told her about Surya Namaskar she looked at me unbelievingly. She couldn't think of doing something which seemed so vigorous. But, because of her faith in me, she agreed to do just one round. Now she does ten rounds of this *asana* and two hours of back-breaking dance every day and is still up and about!

Technique

- STEP I– Stand straight with feet close together. Join hands in front of your chest.

- STEP II– Inhaling, raise arms up, fully stretching the body, bending backward.

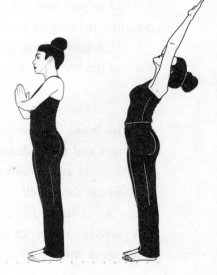

- STEP III- Exhaling, bend forward to place hands on the floor to the outside of your feet. (Initially you may bend your knees to assume the correct posture.)

- STEP IV- Inhaling, extend the right leg backward while bringing down the hips to rest on the left heel. The face should be turned upward.

- STEP V - Exhaling, lift the hips high up while taking the left foot back to join the right one. Keep head down and in between the arms.

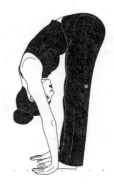

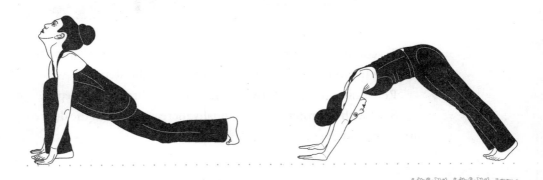

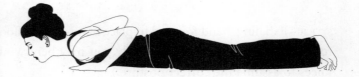

- STEP VI- Retaining the breath outside, lower yourself down to let the entire body except the pelvis rest on the floor.

- STEP VII- Drop the stomach on to the floor. Inhaling, raise head and then the rest of the trunk up. Navel downward should remain on the floor.

- STEP VIII- Same as step V

- STEP IX- Same as step IV

- STEP X- Same as step III

- STEP XI- Same as step II

- STEP XII- Same as step I

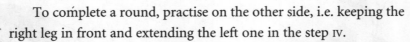

To complete a round, practise on the other side, i.e. keeping the right leg in front and extending the left one in the step IV.

Remember to bring forward the right foot first in the step IX.

Start with 2-3 rounds and gradually increase them till the desired number is attained.

SHASHANK BHUJANGASANA

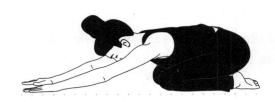 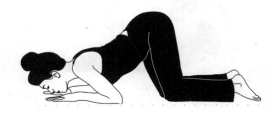

Technique

- Sit in Vajrasan
- Raise arms up.
- Take a deep breath
- Exhaling, bend forward and place the head and the forearms on the ground.
- Inhaling, slide forward keeping the body as close to the floor as possible.

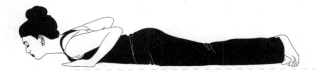

- When the body is fully stretched, move it upward from the waist, arching the back and stretching till the arms are straight.

- Hold the posture for a few seconds.

  - Exhaling, lift the hips and sit back on the heels, keeping the head on the floor.

- Inhaling, slide again.

- Continue the whole process in a smooth movement 7 to 10 times.

DRUT HALASAN

Technique

- Lie down on the back with arms at the sides of the body and palms facing down.

- Take a deep breath and exhale

- Holding the breath out, lift the legs up.

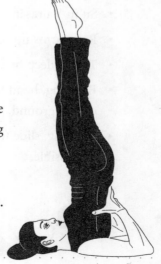

- Taking them above your head try to touch the ground with your feet.

- Quickly take the legs back to the starting position and sit up.

- Quickly bend forward to hold the toes, keeping the head down.

- Return to the starting position and do the exercise continuously for few more rounds.

- Starting with five rounds increase the number to ten.

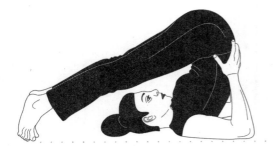
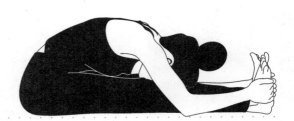

Spot

Slimmers

Chapter II

The yogic exercises of the previous chapter affect the entire body and reduce fat from all over. But, unfortunately, fat is not always distributed evenly. Guided mostly by hereditary factors, it accumulates at certain body parts such as the hips, waist, arms or thighs, while other parts remain slim. For people with such tendencies, reducing evenly may lead to unwanted consequences. For example people with narrow hips and thick waist, wanting to reduce their waistline, may also lose inches from the hips and end up having a slim but straight body without a pleasing contour. One may also lose fat unnecessarily from the face and look haggard. Therefore tackling a problem area alone with specific yogic exercises is a better option.

PADA HASTASANA (FOR THE STOMACH)

Technique

- Stand straight with feet joined.

- Inhaling, raise arms up.

- Exhaling, quickly bend forward to touch the toes.

- Inhaling, quickly stand up with arms raised.

- Repeat ten times, gradually increasing the number to twenty.

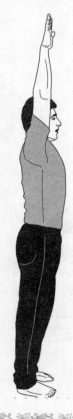

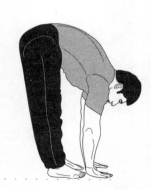

TRIKON 1 — (WAIST AND THIGHS)

Technique

- Stand straight with legs wide apart and arms stretched out sidesways. Take a deep breath.

- Exhaling, and bending the right knee, bend to the right and touch the right foot.

- Bring the left arm down and hold it parallel to the ground, turning the face up. Inhaling, return to the starting position.

- Repeat on the other side to complete one round.

- Practice five to seven rounds, increasing the number to ten.

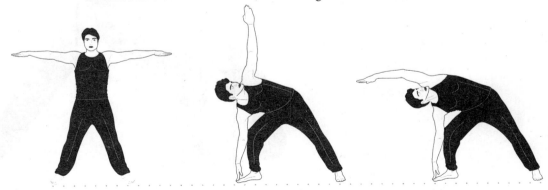

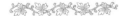

TRIKON II — (WAIST, THIGHS AND BACK)

Technique

- Stand straight with legs apart.
- Hold hands behind the back.
- Take a deep breath.
- Exhaling, and bending the right knee, bend forward to touch the knee with the nose.
- Hold the posture for a few seconds.
- Inhaling, return to the starting position.
- Practise on the other side.
- Repeat five to seven times initially and increase it to ten rounds.

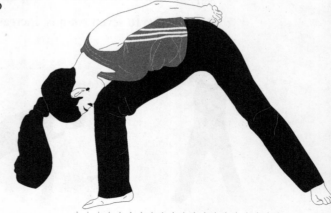

TRIKON III — (WAIST)

Technique

- Stand with legs apart
- Exhaling, bend to the left, sliding the left hand down the left leg, while moving the right hand up on the right side of the trunk.
- Inhaling, return to starting position.
- Practise on the other side.
- Repeat ten times.

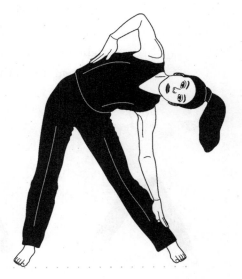

TRIKON IV — (STOMACH AND WAIST)

Technique

- Stand with legs apart and arms stretched out sideways.

- Take a deep breath.

- Exhaling, bend forward.

- Holding the breath, twist to the left from the waist and touch the left foot with the right hand while turning the head up from the left side to look at the left hand. Quickly swing to the right and touch the right foot with the left hand while the face is turned up on the right side.

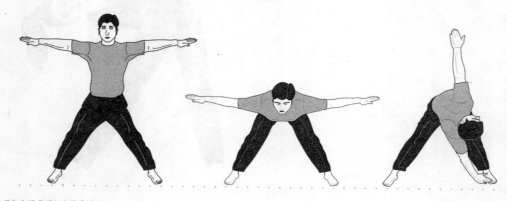

- Quickly return to the body's forward bent position.

- Inhaling, straighten up to the starting position.

- Repeat five times, gradually increasing the number to ten.

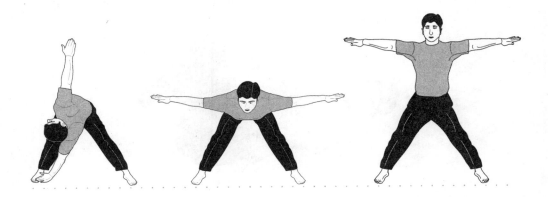

SIDE ROLLING — (HIPS AND WAIST)

Technique

- Spread a thin sheet on a hard floor.

- Lie down on your back.

- Clasp your fingers and place hands under the head.

- Bend the knees and bring them up on to your chest.

- Keeping the upper part of the body firmly on the ground, twist the lower part to the left and let the joined knees touch the floor.

- Immediately swing to the right to let the knees touch the floor on the right side.

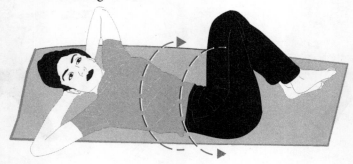

- Swing again to the left.

- Roll from side to side continuously 10-15 times.

- The number can be increased to 40-50.

BACK ROLLING — (BACK)

Technique

- Sit on your haunches.

- Wrap arms around the legs.

- Rock your body forward and backward on the floor 10 – 15 times.

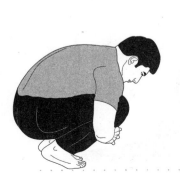 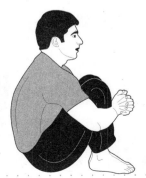 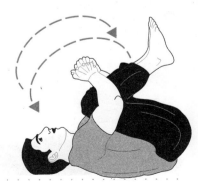

MERU AKARSHANASANA — (THIGHS)

Technique

- Lie on your right side with the upper part of the body propped up supported by the right arm.

- Inhaling, lift the left leg as high as possible and hold the big toe with the left hand.

- Exhaling return to the starting position.

- Practise ten times.

- Turn to the left and repeat.

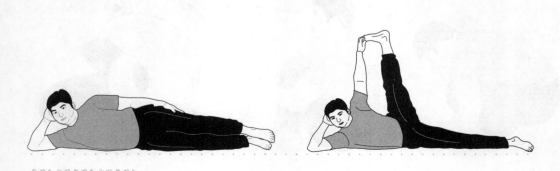

SPOT SLIMMERS

HASTA ANGUSHTASANA — (THIGHS AND ARMS)

- Lie down on your right side with the arms stretched above the head with hands joined.

- Inhaling, raise the left leg.

- Move the left hand and touch the toe.

- Hold the posture for a few seconds.

- Exhaling, return to the starting position moving the limbs slowly.

- Practise ten times.

- Turn to your left side and repeat.

- Hold the posture and breathe normally 20 times.

- Inhaling, sit up.

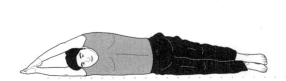
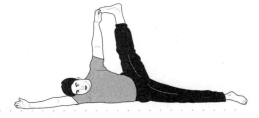
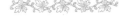

Obesity caused by other factors

"I just have to look at food to put on weight", moan many an obese person. Obviously they do not know that obesity is not always the result of overeating. It can also be the result of a systemic failure — the most common being a sluggish thyroid.

The thyroid gland, situated at the base of the neck secretes a hormone called thyroxine, which is released into the blood stream to regulate the pace of chemical activities in the body. The more the hormone in the blood, the faster are the chemical activities and the more are the calories burnt. When the amount of thyroxine exceeds its upper limit, it becomes a clinical problem called hyper-thyroidism. A patient of this condition remains painfully thin, no matter how high the calory intake. The exact opposite happens when the thyroid becomes sluggish. The person tends to put on weight even with an extremely low-calorie diet.

Generally, altroxine is prescribed for a thyroid problem which eliminates the symptoms for a while. But, a weak body part can only become weaker with time, so it is with this gland. So thyroid secretes less and less thyroxine, which calls for an increase in the dose of the medicine again and again. Too much of altroxine can affect the system adversely, especially the heart. Once the heart is damaged

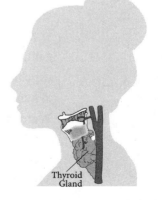

Thyroid
Gland

not much can be done to normalise the condition. A person with a heart problem is not allowed to practise *asanas* necessary to cure hypothyroidism; and the heart condition cannot be improved when one is taking altroxine. At the same time the medicine cannot be withdrawn as that can throw the entire system out of gear. And thus the patient becomes totally dependent on these harmful drugs for life. Hence the abnormal condition of the thyroid should be cured before it is too late. With sustained *yoga* practise many have managed to arrest their condition and some have even reversed it.

The normal range of thyroxine secretion is wide. As long as it remains within this range, even if it is the lowest, medical science considers the thyroid function as normal. But the metabolism of such a person is slow and the weight gain high.

Sluggishness of kidneys, lungs or the heart can also lead to weight gain, though the weight is that of water alone. The body is constantly expelling water from the system as urine, sweat, and through breath. When these organs become weak, they cannot do this job effectively. Water accumulates in the body, causing water retention or oedema.

Diet deficiency is yet another cause of obesity. After all, even the thyroid requires proper food to remain healthy and function well. Missing meals and starving can only produce unwelcome

consequences. Calcium and iron deficiencies too can lead to obesity.

The following yogic *asanas* strengthen these major glands. Organ metabolism increases; stored fat gets burnt; accumulated water is eliminated; and the body is brought to a proper shape.

SARVANGASANA

This *asana* stimulates the thyroid gland by exerting pressure on it and drawing extra blood to the area.

Technique

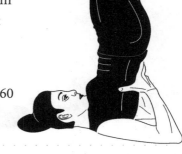

- Lie down on your back

- Bend the legs and bring them on to your chest. Holding the rib cage with both your hands, assume shoulder stand position. The body from shoulder down should remain vertical, almost 90 degree to the floor.

- Breathe normally.

- Starting with ten breaths gradually go up to 60 breaths.

- To return, first bend the legs and slowly lower yourself.
- The head should remain firmly on the floor.
- Sarvangasana should be followed by Supta Vajrasana after a short rest.

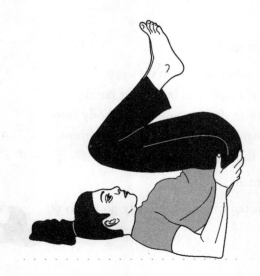

SUPTA VAJRASANA

Technique

- Sit in Vajrasana
- Arching the back, bend backward and with the support of your arms, lower your head to the ground. The corner of the head should be placed on the floor. Place hands on your thighs and breathe normally.
- Starting with five breaths go up to 30.
- Taking support of the arms sit up.
- Unfold the legs.
- Lie down to rest.

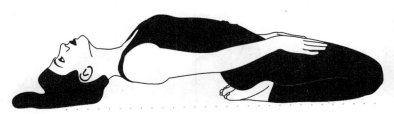

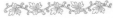

YOGA MUDRA ASANA

Technique

- Sit in Vajrasana.

- Make fists with your hands and place them on the thighs pressing against your body.

- Take a deep breath.

- Exhaling, bend forward and place your head on the floor.

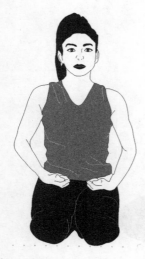
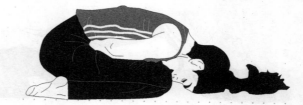

SHALABHASANA

Technique

- Lie on your stomach with the face down.
- Place hands under the thighs, palms turned down.
- Inhale.
- Lift legs up without bending the knees.
- Hold the posture as long as comfortable.
- Exhaling, lower the legs and relax.
- Repeat five times.

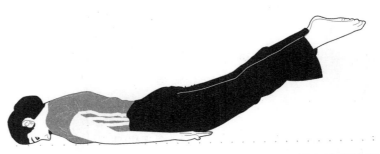

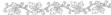

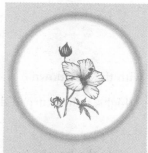

Toners

A well-toned body is not only beautiful, but is healthy and youthful. Unexercised muscles lose their firmness and become slack. The force of gravity then pulls them downwards making them hang. The features become shapeless and unattractive. The skin under the eyes become loose; the jawline disappears; busts sag; arms become flabby and the abdomen protrudes. It can only worsen with age. It is worse with overweight people after they lose the extra weight. As the fat dissolves, the overstretched skin loses its support. It hangs, becoming more prone to the gravity's downward pull. The firmness of each muscle can be maintained to a great extent with appropriate yogasanas. Though yoga's effect is always positive, even dramatic at some stages, it should be adopted as a preventive measure for the best result.

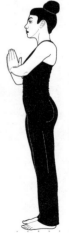

SIMHASANA

This *asana* firms up the facial muscles including the delicate ones under the eyes; jawline and the neck.

Technique

- Sit in Vajrasana with knees apart.

- Place hands on the floor in between the knees pointing towards you.

- Bend the head backward stretching the neck fully.

- Open your mouth wide, extend the tongue fully; cross eyes and look up at the middle of the eyebrows.

- Take a deep breath through the nose.

- Make the sound aaaaaaa.............. while you breathe out from the mouth.

- Repeat ten times.

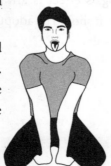
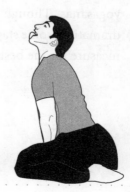

Rope pulling

The muscles and ligaments in and around the busts are exercised and toned by this *asana*.

Technique

- Sit on the floor with legs stretched in front.

- Place the hands on the legs.

- Lift the right arm up with the palm open. Close fingers and clench them into a fist as if you are holding a rope

- Applying a little resistance, pull the imaginary rope down bringing the hand down to the right leg.

- Repeat on the left side.

- Pull rope in a quick and continuous fashion.

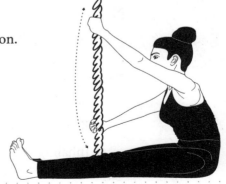

CHOPPING WOOD

The benefits are the same as the previous *asanas*.

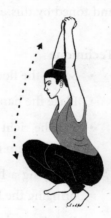

Technique

- Sit on your haunches.

- Interlock the fingers.

- Inhaling, lift your hands up and with sudden force, bring the hands down as if chopping wood.

- Repeat ten times.

NAUKASANA

This *asana* tones up the abdominal muscles.

Technique

- Lie down on your back.

- Keep the arms beside your body.

- Inhaling, lift your head and legs above the ground, arms stretched in front.

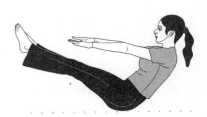

- The head, hands and feet should remain at the same level.

- Hold the posture for as long as possible.

- Exhaling, return to the starting position.

CHAKKI CHALANA

The continuous forward and backward movement of the body tones the stomach while exercising and strengthening the arms as well.

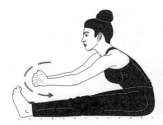

Technique

- Sit with legs in front.

- Interlock the fingers.

- Inhale.

- Exhaling, bend forward while moving the hands clockwise.

- Inhaling, bend backward and bring the hand in anti-clockwise to complete a circle.

- The action imitates grinding a mill.

- Practise ten times in one direction then ten times in the other direction.

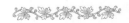

NAUKA SANCHALAN

The benefits are the same as the previous one.

Technique

- Sitting in the same position as the previous *asana* imitate rowing a boat

- Exhale while bending forward

- Inhale while pulling the hands in and bending backward.

- Repeat ten times.

- Now move the arms in the opposite direction.

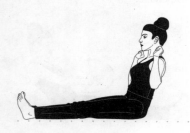 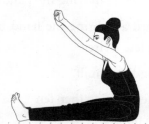 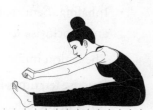

Ashwa Sanchalan

The benefits are the same as the previous one.

Technique

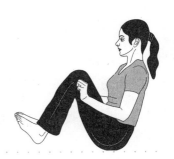

- Sit on the floor.

- Bend the legs and keep the feet flat in front on the floor.

- Make fists with your hands and hold them outside the knees.

- Lift your feet up and balance on your hips.

- Inhaling, bend backwards while straightening your legs and moving them upward.

- Exhaling, return to the starting position.

- Moving quickly, repeat the whole process ten times.

- The hands remain near the knees while the arms straighten and bend with the legs.

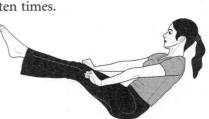

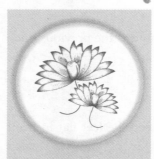

Glandular
Glamour

CHAPTER V

A well-known beautician comments 'glamour is glandular'. How true! Many of the beauty problems, especially of the skin and hair are only the result of malfunctioning glands.

The softness of the skin is maintained by sebum, a lubricant, secreted by a set of glands called sebaceous glands. They are distributed all over the skin including the scalp. If these glands are overactive, the skin becomes thick and oily with large open pores. Dirt clogs the pores and traps the oil inside, creating a source of infection, which is the main reason for pimples, blackheads and whiteheads. The hair too becomes oily and limp with the excessive oil secreted in the scalp. At the same time underproduction of sebum results in dry hair and dry skin which in turn gives rise to the most dreaded enemy of beauty—wrinkles.

The skin owes its rosy tint to the red colour of the blood. The more the red cells in the blood, the redder is its colour and the pinker is the skin. These red blood cells are made from iron and the absorption of this mineral from food depends on the health of the liver. An unhealthy liver cannot discharge its duty well and anaemia occurs. The skin assumes a pale ghostly look.

Even the eyes lose their charm, no matter how beautifully they are shaped.

In every human body, both male and female hormones are secreted. Excessive male hormones give rise to excessive hair growth, while excess female hormones lead to scanty hair.

Too much thyroid hormone also leads to profuse hair and too little results in thin and lacklustre ones. A sluggish thyroid thickens the body, leads to dry itchy skin and puffy face; while an overactive gland can make the eyes bulge and look ugly.

Thyroid is controlled by the pituitary gland. Only an exact amount of its thyrotropic hormone keeps the thyroid function normal. An erratic pituitary obviously makes the thyroid erratic too. Other glands are also affected because pituitary is the master of them all. Pituitary itself affects one's appearance. If it produces too much growth hormones—even during the middle age years—the hands, feet and jaw start growing bigger, sometimes becoming enormous. Apart from making the person look grotesque, it also hastens the ageing process and turns a youth into an old man in a matter of months.

A handsome man who aspired to become a film star developed this problem. Soon he turned into a giant of a man with enlarged,

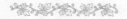

ugly features. Ultimately, he was reduced to doing negative roles in horror movies in Bombay. I am told, he is dead now. He was only in his forties.

Pituitary too is not completely independent. It is controlled by hypothalamus which in turn is influenced by the state of our mind. And thus sound mental health and perfect glandular function are essential for perfect beauty. The following yogasanas, along with meditation, normalise the glandular function.

SURYANAMASKAR

Suryanamaskar also is excellent for the sebaceous glands. Ideally, 10-12 rounds of it should be practised everyday facing the morning sun. The perspiration should then be rubbed back into the body to cure skin problems.

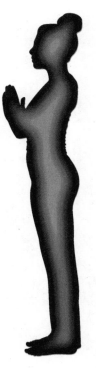

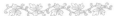

Paschimottanasana — (Liver)

- Sit on the floor with legs stretched in front.

- Inhaling, lift arms up.

- Exhaling, bend forward and hold the toes. If that is not possible, hold any part of the legs below the knees.

- Breathe normally, keeping the head down.

- Hold the posture for one minute or so.

- Inhaling, lift arms and straighten the body.

- Exhaling, bring hands down to the legs.

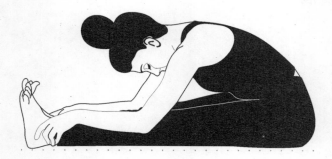

TOLANGULASANA — (LIVER)

- Assume Padmasana.
- Keeping the legs locked, lie down on your back.
- Put hands under the buttocks
- Supporting your body with the forearms rise and lift the legs.
- Inhale and bend the head forward, chin pressing against the chest.
- Hold the posture as long as you are comfortable.
- Lift head, exhale, and return to the starting position.
- Repeat five times.

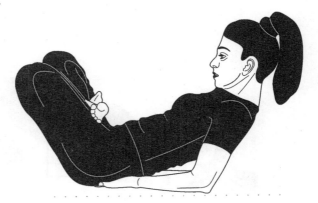

KANDHRASANA — (ALL GLANDS)

- Lie down on your back.

- Bend legs and place feet flat beside the hips.

- Hold the ankles.

- Take a deep breath.

- Lift the pelvic area up while the head and shoulders remain on the ground.

- Hold the posture for a while.

- Exhaling, lower yourself.

- Repeat five times.

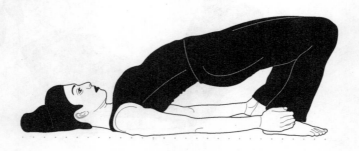

BHUMI PADA MASTAKASANA — (PITUITARY)

- Sit in Vajrasana.
- Place hands on the floor in front of you at a distance of about two feet.
- Rise to hold the torso parallel to the ground.
- Place the head on the floor on a folded blanket.
- Lift the body to a triangular position.
- Take your hands back and hold the right wrist with the left hand.
- Hold the posture for a comfortable duration.
- Lower the body to Shashankasana.
- After two minutes lie down in Shavasana.

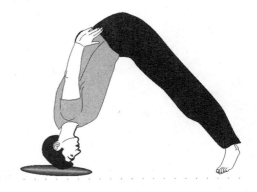

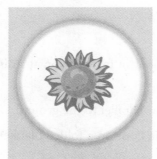

The
Ultimate
Anti-Agers

According to *hatha yoga*, *mudras* and *bandhas* are the best anti-agers. It says:

महामुद्रा महाबंधो महावेधश्च खेचरी।
उडीयानं मूलबंधश्च बंधो जालंधराभिधः॥

करणी विपरीताख्या वज्रोली शक्तिचालनम्।
इंद हि मुद्रादशकं जरामरणनाशनम्॥

Literaly translated it means, Mahamudra, Mahabandha, Mahaveda, Khechari, Uddiyana, Moolabandha, Jalandhara Bandha, Vipareeta Karani, Vajroli and Shakti Chalanam — these ten *mudras* destroy old age and death.

Mudras and *bandhas* are an integral and important part of *hatha yoga*. Though they resemble the normal yogasanas, their functions are different. *Asanas* aim to release the energy blocks while *bandhas* lock the energy inside the body and *mudras* channelise it and send it to specific body parts. *Asanas*, *mudras* and *bandhas* work in unison to give the desired results.

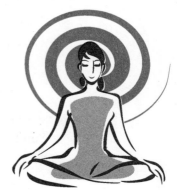

MAHA MUDRA

- Sit down with legs stretched in the front.

- Bend the left leg and press the heel against the perineum.

- Fold the tongue (Khechari)

- Take a deep breath

- Exhaling, bend forward and hold the right big toe with both hands.

- As you inhale slowly, lift the head back.

- Crossing the eyes, look up to the point in between the eyebrows.

- Contract the perineum.

- Hold your breath and the posture for a comfortable duration.

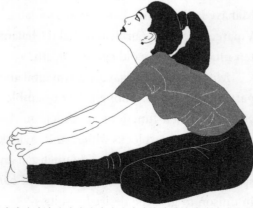

End the *mudra* in the following manner:

- Close your eyes.
- Relax the contraction of the perineum.
- Bring back the head to its normal position and exhale.
- Relax for a while, then repeat.
- Practise five times.

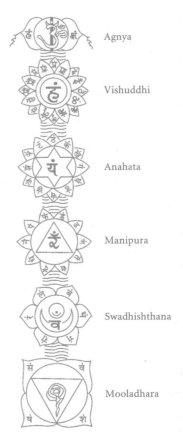

Thereafter, practice three times with the right leg bent.

In the final posture you may rotate your consciousness over the *chakras* while repeating their names mentally – i.e. *agnya, vishuddhi, anahata, manipura, swadhishthana* and *mooladhara.*

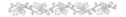

JALANDHARA BANDHA

- Assume Padmasana (lotus pose) or just cross your legs.

- Keep the hands on the knees with palms facing down.

- Breathe in—slow and deep.

- Retaining the breath inside, bend your head forward till the chin touches the chest.

- Straightening the arms, lift the shoulders.

- Hold the posture till comfortable.

- Lower the shoulders to their normal position.

- Lift head and slowly exhale.

- Relax for around a minute before repeating the *bandha*.

- Practise five times.

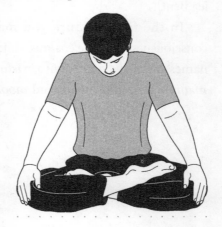

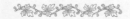

UDDIYANA BANDHA

- Sit on a cushion and assume Padmasana (lotus pose).

- Place hands on the respective knees.

- Take a deep breath.

- Exhale through the mouth with lips slightly pursed. Bending the head, lift shoulders as in Jalandhara Bandha.

- Pull in the stomach as much as possible as if to touch the spine.

- Hold the posture as long as comfortable.

- Relax the stomach.

- Release the shoulder lock.

- Lift head to its normal position and then inhale.

- Wait for a minute before repeating the *bandha*.

- Practise five times.

- Uddiyana Bandha has a variation which is much easier for stiff bodied practitioners and it is done in a standing position.

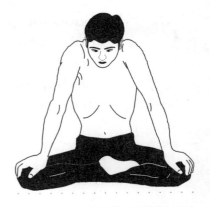

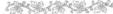

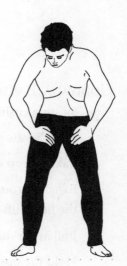

STANDING UDDIYANA

- Stand with feet apart.

- Bend and place hands on the thighs.

- Keeping the spine straight, bend the knees a little.

- Take a deep breath and practise the *bandha* the same way as the original one.

MOOLABANDHA

This *bandha* involves contraction of the *Mooladhara Chakra* – the lowest of the six energy centers of the spinal cord. *Mooladhara*, located in the perineum near the tip of the tailbone is a very important chakra as it is considered to be the abode of *kundalini* – the source of *prana* (vital force) and power. Contraction of this point releases *prana* which spreading all over the body relaxes and rejuvenates the worn-out body cells.

Technique

- Sit in a meditative pose such as Padmasana, Siddhasana or Sukhasana.

- Place hands on the knees with the tips of the index fingers touching the thumbs.

- Perform Jalandhara Bandha.

- Concentrate on the *Mooladhara Chakra*.

- Contract it partially and hold it for a little while; contract a little more and hold.

- Continue in this position till the area is fully contracted.

- Hold the contraction for as long as possible while breathing normally.

- Repeat five times.

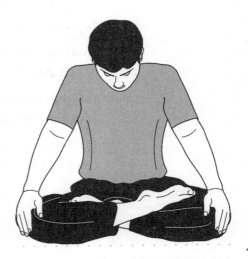

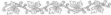

MAHA BANDHA

Maha Bandha literally means the great lock. This technique combines all the three *bandhas* and gives the benefits of each *chakra* in a magnified way. It effectively averts the decaying process of the body.

Technique

- Sit in Padmasana.

- Take a deep breath slowly and exhale through the mouth. Try to expel as much air as possible.

- Bend the head forward to perform Jalandhara Bandh.

- Contract the perineum as in Moola Bandha.

- Pull the stomach in and perform Uddiyana Bandha.

- Hold the posture as long as comfortable.

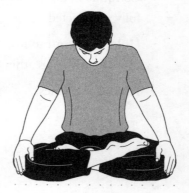

- Release the perineum, then the stomach, then the shoulders and finally lift your head and inhale.

- Relax for a minute or so.

- Repeat five times.

VAJROLI

This *mudra* is said to prevent and cure impotence and prostrate gland problems.

Technique

- Sit in a meditative pose.

- Relax the body.

- Concentrate on the urethra.

- Take a deep breath and contract it.

- Hold the posture for a comfortable duration.

- Exhale and release the contraction.

- Repeat 3-5 times and gradually increase the number to ten.

Khechari

According to yoga, *amrit*—the nectar of youth is produced in the *bindu chakra* which is located at the top corner of the head. When the nectar drops, it flows down through the throat and is consumed by the heat of the lower *chakras* and is lost. But when its passage in the nasal cavity is blocked, entering the blood stream it circulates in the body bestowing amazing benefits to the practitioner. It is said that a yogi who can keep his tongue even for half a second in the nasal cavity, is freed from diseases, old age and death.

Traditionally, the tongue is elongated for this purpose. The process is complicated and time consuming and needs to be started early in life. Portions from the lower surface of the tongue are cut systematically from time to time. The tongue is then exercised and milked regularly, to lengthen it. Eventually it becomes long enough for its tip to be inserted into the nasal passage from the throat when it is turned backward.

One may not be able to practise Khechari Mudra in the manner mentioned above, but even by folding the tongue backward with its underside against the palate, one can get immense benefit.

MAHABHEDA MUDRA

Technique

- Sit with legs outstretched.

- Do Khechari Mudra.

- Take a deep breath.

- Exhaling, bend forward and hold the big toe.

- Perform Jalandhara, Uddiyana and Moola Bandh.

- Hold the posture till comfortable.

- Release Moola, Uddiyana and Jalandhara Bandhas.

- Inhale.

- Practise three rounds.

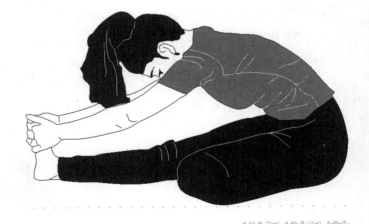

VIPREET KARANI MUDRA

The inverted posture of this *mudra* makes the body fluids flow down to the head and mix with the nectar of the *bindu chakra* which is then assimilated into the system. The meaning of Vipareet Karani is that which reverses.

Technique

- Lie down on your back.

- Lift the body up from above the waist.

- Support the trunk with your hands.

- Straighten the legs to a vertical position.

- The trunk should be held at 45 degree to the floor.

- Breathe normally and hold the posture for a comfortable duration.

- Slowly return to the starting position.

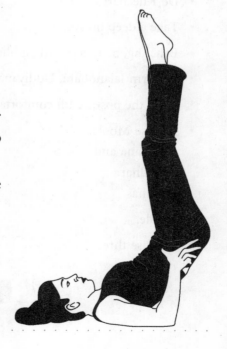

Shakti Chalana

Shakti is energy and *chalana* means moving. In this *mudra*, energy is made to move and gather intensity and momentum.

Technique

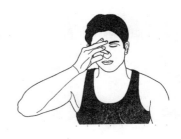

- Take a deep breath through the right nostril by blocking the left nostril.

- Retaining the breath, contract the perineum.

- Hold the posture for as long as possible.

- Exhale deeply.

- Drop the head to perform Jalandhara and Uddiyan Bandhas.

- Perform *nauli* by isolating the two vertical rectus abdomini muscles and rotating them ten times clockwise and ten times anti-clockwise.

- Release Uddiyan, then Jalandhara.

- Lift your head and inhale.

- After a short rest, repeat.

- Gradually increase the number to five.

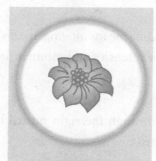

Radiance
Enhancer

Oxygen is known to be a great beauty enhancer. The glow it imparts to the skin cannot be matched by any other beauty aid. And its effect is instantaneous, as can be seen after a brisk long walk in the open — the eyes sparkle and the cheeks look flushed — a fact that has led to the mushrooming of many oxygen parlours all over the world.

But, the easy availability of oxygen does not guarantee adequate absorption of this gas into the system; or else no asthmatic or chronic heavy smoker would gasp for breath. Absorption of oxygen depends on the condition of the respiratory system and the mode of breathing.

The lungs are spongy structures with innumerable tiny air sacs, called alvioli, which expand with inhalation to receive the fresh air and contract during exhalation to squeeze the carbon dioxide out. The air passages are lined with tiny hair, called cilia, which filter the impurities from the air and sweep them up and out of the body. If the respiratory system is unhealthy, producing excessive mucus, the cilia get drowned and cannot do their job. They also get paralysed into inaction by nicotine smoke. And thus, suspended particles enter the lungs unhindered. They clog the tiny air passages and scar

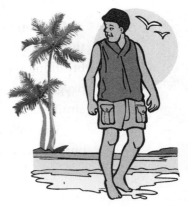

the lung tissues. The scarred delicate air sacs lose their elasticity and cannot contract well enough with exhalation. Carbon dioxide gets trapped in them, preventing the entry of oxygen.

Superficial breathing, using only a little of the upper part of the lungs, also prevents adequate oxygen supply. In habitual shallow breathings, the lower part of the lungs and the diaphragm are never used. These unexercised parts lose their strength and become weak and can barely move. Stale air accumulates there giving rise to ill health and pale appearance.

Fast breathing is as incorrect as shallow breathing as time is required for the oxygen to be transferred to the blood, and carbon di oxide from the blood to the lungs. Hence, slow deep breathing, and a clean respiratory system are essential for proper utilization of this wonderful bounty of nature. Yoga exercises and strengthens the breathing apparati and encourages correct breathing. Thus optimum oxygenation of the system to enhance one's health and beauty is ensured.

The following *asana* and *pranayama* are excellent for that purpose. (In case of an ailment seek expert advise).

Matsyasana

This is one of the best *asanas* for the lungs. It expands the ribcage and encourages deep respiration.

Technique

- Sit in Padmasana.

- Arching the back, bend backwards. Supporting yourself with the arms, lower the body till the head touches the ground.

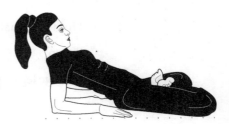

- Place the corner of the head on a folded blanket.

- Hold your toes.

- Breathe normally.

- Hold the posture for as long as required.

- Return to the starting position.

- Unfold the legs and lie down in Shavasana.

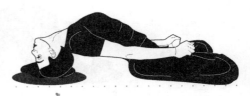

People who cannot sit in Padmasana can practise Matsyasana in the following manner :

Technique

- Sit on the floor with legs stretched in front.
- Bend the left leg and place the foot on the right leg.
- Bend backward as in the previous method.
- Hold the final posture for half the desired duration.
- Sit up.
- Change legs and repeat on the other side for the same duration.

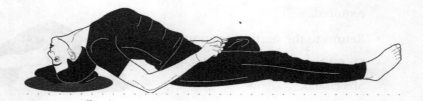

Some people have such stiff bodies that they can hardly bend their legs. They can follow the simplest version.

Technique

- Sit on the floor with legs stretched in front.
- Simply bending backwards with arched back, lower the head to the floor.
- Place the hands on your thighs and breathe normally for the desired duration.

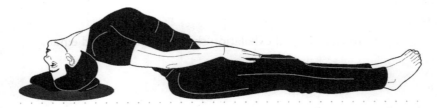

BHASTRIKA

This *pranayama* not only removes the accumulated stagnant gases from the lungs and fills them with fresh air, it also exercises and strengthens the respiratory muscles.

Technique

- Sit in meditation pose.

- Keep the left hand on the left knee in *gyana mudra*.

- Place the index and middle fingers of the right hand on the space in between the eyebrows.

- Close the right nostril with the thumb and breathe 20 times rapidly like bellowing through the left nostril.

- Closing the left nostril with the ring finger repeat the same with the right nostril. Remove the hand from the nose and breathe in the same manner simultaneously through both the nostrils.

- Inhalation and exhalation should be forced and equal.

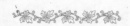

RADIANCE ENHANCER

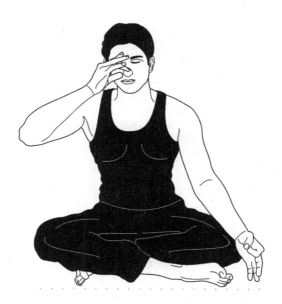

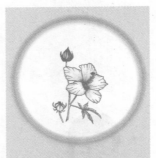

The

Sparkler

Only a clean system can lead to a clean glowing skin. As a white balloon filled with black water cannot look white, the skin cells (which are like tiny translucent balloons) with dirty fluid inside cannot but look dirty.

Pollutants are constantly entering out body through food, water and air. Although the body has its own mechanism to discard harmful foreign matter, it cannot do its job effectively when pollutants exceed its capacity to deal with them. These pollutants are then sent to body cells, including those of the skin to be stored there permanently. Half a pound of unwanted chemicals alone are found to accumulate in one's body every year.

Removing all the toxins from the body is not a very easy job. Long fasts, a fruit diet and intake of gallons of water are some of the recommended measures. But the quickest and the most effective method to detox is yoga. *Pranayama* removes the gaseous toxins, while for the solid ones nothing is better than yogic *shatkriya* called *Guru Shankha Prakshyalana* — *Guru* meaning major, *Shankha* is a conch, and *Prakshyalana* means washing. Here, the intestine, with all its nooks and corners is compared to a conch shell, which is rather difficult to clean.

Guru Shankha Prakshyalana is generally practised once a year before or after winter. It should not be attempted in hard summer, severe winter or during the rains. The *kriya* involves drinking a huge amount of water

and removing the accumulated waste from the intestine. The entire process takes about four to five hours to complete.

This cleaning technique not only scrubs the digestive tract—a major manufacturer of toxins itself—clean, but the saline water circulating all over the body draws out chemicals and other dirty substances from the body cells to the blood stream which are then thrown out of the system by the eliminating organs. With all the pollutants gone from the body, the skin acquires a fresh and clean look with often a pearly transluscence.

Technique
(To be practised strictly under the guidance of an expert)

Heat up thirty glasses of water. Take out six glasses from it and keep them in another container. Add 3 tsp of clean salt to it and mix well. Quickly drink three glasses and perform the following *asanas*, eight times each as in *Laghoo Shankh Prakshalana* (for details, see author's book *Yoga for Busy People*).

1. Tadasana
2. Triyaka Tadasana
3. Kati Chakrasana
4. Triyak Bhujangasana
5. Udarakh.

TADASANA

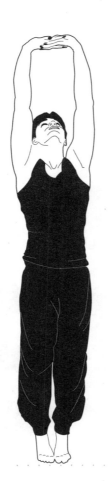

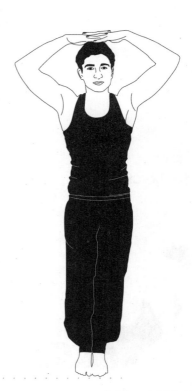

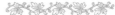

TRIYAKA
TADASANA

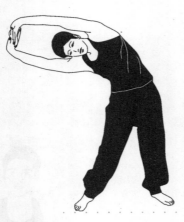

KATI
CHAKRASANA

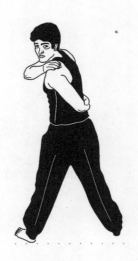

TRIYAK
BHUJANGASANA

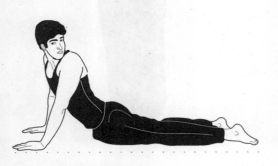

UDARAKH

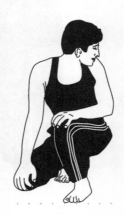

Drink another two glasses quickly, and again practise the *asanas*.
Repeat the whole process once more.

Go to the toilet and clear the bowel.

Normally one has a clear motion at this point. But if you don't feel the urge after this round, practise the following *asanas*:

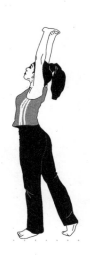

(i) Walking Tadasana – Stand on your toes with arms stretched straight above your head. Stretch your body and walk about for a while.

(ii) Rolling – Lie down on the ground with feet close together. Stretching the arms above your head, join hands. Roll on.

(iii) Kali Asana – Sit on your haunches. Move knees apart. Keeping the elbows on the knees place thumbs under the chin and turn your face up. Maintain the posture for some time. You can rock forward and backward on your feet. Almost certainly you will feel the urge to pass bowel.

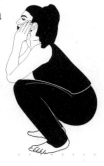

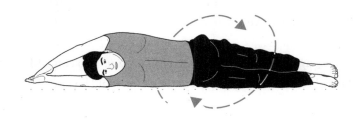

From now on drink two glasses of warm saline water (less salty than the first six glasses), practise the same *asanas* the same number of times and pass bowel.

Continue the cycle till you pass clear water. Now, there is nothing left in the intestine.

Practise *kunjal* and *neti* (see *Yoga for Busy People*)

Lie down in Shavasana and rest for forty-five minute.

After 45 minutes, you have to eat a special *khichdi* which has to be prepared fresh by somebody else during your resting time. At least 150 gms of ghee (clarified butter) is then added to this saltless and extra soft preparation of rice and lentil. You should eat as much *khichdi* as you possibly can—even to the point of overstuffing your stomach. You must finish eating within half an hour. After the meal, relax for three hours, but do not sleep—you can move about without exerting yourself.

During this time you must not drink any water. If you feel too thirsty, you can put half a teaspoon of water in your mouth just to wet the tongue and throat. After three hours, it is essential to drink one or two glasses of water.

In the evening, again have freshly prepared *khichdi*. You can add a little salt but no *ghee*. Next day breakfast and lunch should be *khichdi* only. For dinner you can have rice and lentil separately prepared, and some boiled vegetables.

In the first week following this *kriya* only rice, lentil and certain vegetables are allowed. Vegetables such as potatoes, carrots, beans, onion, garlic, ginger etc. are not permitted. Other prohibited foods are fruits, milk, milk products, salads, nuts, alcohol, drugs, sour things and non-vegetarian food.

In the second week you can eat everything except chillies, alcohol, non-vegetarian and rich spicy food. After two weeks, you can gradually go back to normal food, though avoiding chillies, non-vegetarian and deep fried food for another two weeks yields the best result.

In yoga, *Guru Shanka Prakshyasana* is considered a major *kriya* which can be likened to a major surgery. Not following its various rules and regulations strictly, can lead to serious problems. Hence, it must be practised under expert supervision, at least the very first time. All the dos and donts attached to this *kriya* often discourage people from practising it. But the benefits of *Guru Shankha Prakshyalan* are so wide and wonderful that one should smilingly bear with the inconveniences. One must remember that nothing comes without a price!

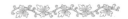

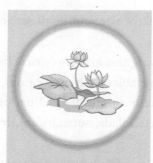

Beauty
Creator

CHAPTER IX

BEAUTY CREATOR

In the popular story of *Alladin and the Magic Lamp*, Alladin rubbed the lamp by mistake. Out came a mighty jinn. The jinn bowed to the little boy and asked 'Master, what is it that you desire? Command, and it shall be yours'. The wonder-struck boy asked for food and lo! In the twinkling of an eye, gold and silver bowls filled with all sorts of delicacies appeared before him. Alladin then wanted to marry the most beautiful princess; a palace to live in; and the enemy army to be vanquished. All his wishes were fulfilled by the jinn in no time at all.

We also have a jinn under our command. It too can get us whatever we want. It is the mightiest of them all. But alas! We never use it. It remains locked in its abode and we do not even attempt to unlock it. The jinn here is our inner mind—the source of all power, which lies buried by the conscious outer one.

Mental power has been used by people the world over from time to time to acquire name, fame, success and wealth. Martial art practitioners use it to defend themselves against armed assailants; saints have used it to cure the lame, blind, deaf and the dumb; and yogis have used it to produce matter from thin air. Surely, we can also use it to create health, youth and beauty for ourselves.

The secret force behind perfect health and beauty, according to yoga, is *prana*—the vital life force that animates the inanimates. By mobilising this energy by our mind we can create wonder. *Prana* is present everywhere—in our body and outside. For the best result both the inner and outer *prana* are used.

INCREASING THE INNER PRANA

Technique

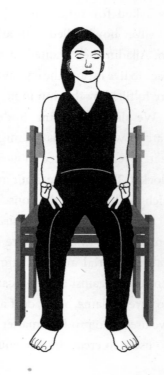

- Sit on a chair with your feet flat on the ground.

- Join the tips of the thumbs with the index fingers in both the hands.

- Place hands on the legs.

- Close your eyes.

- Inhale and imagine golden *prana* being sucked into your right leg from the ground through the bones and spreading all over the leg.

- Practise it a few times.

- In this manner practise it for all the body parts in the following sequence—left leg, right arm, left arm, trunk and head.

- Then take all the *prana* to *mooladhara chakra* near the tip of the tailbone.

- Visualise your body glowing with perfect health.

- Open your eyes.

MOBILISING THE INNER PRANA

Technique
- Sit in a meditative pose or lie down in Shavasana.

- Close your eyes.

- Concentrate on your breath.

- It should be natural and spontaneous.

- Mentally repeat—health, youth, beauty for a few minutes.

- Now breathe in the following manner:

  - Inhale to the count of 7.

  - Hold breath inside for 1 count

- Exhale to the count of 7.
  - Hold breath outside for 1 count.
- Continue for a few minutes.
- Change the ratio to 6:3 - 6:3 i.e. inhale to the count of 6; retain to the count of 3; exhale to the count of 6 and retain to the count of 3. Breathe normally after a few minutes concentrating on the natural flow.
- Shift your concentration to *mooladhara chakra* – the source of *prana*.
- Visualise this vital force as a golden light.
- The *prana* has to be taken to *agnya chakra* – the point in between the eyebrows – via *manipura* and *visuddhi* in the following manner for distribution.
- With inhalation bring *prana* from *mooladhara* to the navel.

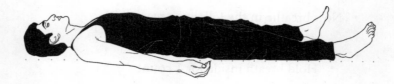

- With exhalation, take your consciousness back to *mooladhara*.

- Repeat 27 times. In the same way take *prana* to the throat from the navel and then to *agnya* from the throat.

The distribution of *prana* to all the body parts is done in the following way:

- Visualise a sun in the centre of the eyebrow and concentrate on it.

- After a while, visualise streaks of light from the sun moving in all direction and flooding each and every tissue of the body.

- Retaining the breath outside, visualise various body parts absorbing the energy; and with inhalation withdraw the rays to the sun.

- Practise for as long as you have the time.

- Then return *prana* to *mooladhara* through the spinal cord.

- Visualise yourself in the desired state – with a smooth and glowing skin.

- Feel rejuvenated from inside.

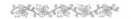

- Externalise your mind.
- Stretch your body.
- Open your eyes.

IN CONJUNCTION WITH PRANAYAMA

This is practised with Nadisodhan Pranayama.

Technique

- Sit in a meditative pose.
- Practise Nadisodhan Pranayama (for details, see author's book *Yoga for Busy People*)
- Visualise a sun at the tip of your nose.
- Inhale golden rays from the sun.
- During retention of breath visualise *prana* spreading all over the body. Visualise individual body parts surrounded by the golden light.
- Exhale smoky impurities which, gradually decreasing, turn colourless on the last round.

BEAUTY CREATOR

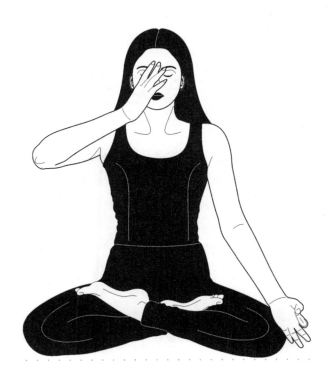

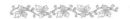

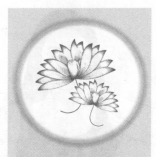

Age
Retarder

The Count of Monte Christo was poisoned and buried by his unfaithful wife. But the Count was not dead. He had only become unconscious. When he regained his consciousness, he found himself locked up in his coffin. Labouring hard, the Count managed to extricate himself from his grave. Coming out to the open, he entered a shop where he chanced to glance at a mirror. He was surprised to see a complete stranger with white hair staring back at him. And suddenly, to the Count's horror, he realised that it was none else but him. He had turned grey overnight!

The above story may be fiction, but not far from the truth. History too has many such examples. Lloyd George—one of the famous Prime Ministers of England—looked prematurely old within hours of hearing that the first World War had broken out. Similar was the fate of Adolf Hitler during the Second World War when Nazi Germany started losing major battles. The bio-clock is found to tick the fastest under stress, speeding up the cell division. Every time, a body cell divides, it loses a little of its long tail till there is no tail left. When the cell can no longer divide itself, it dies, never to be replaced. And thus the body degenerates and ages. It has also been found that the clock ticks at a slower rate when a person is relaxed—the deeper the relaxation, the slower is the rate of ticking. Yogic relaxation techniques induce the deepest possible rest, while certain other yogic practices promote better tissue regeneration. Thus the

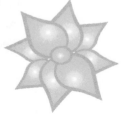

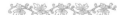

difference between body's degeneration and regeneration is minimised resulting in slow ageing.

Though all yogic practices induce relaxation, *Yoganidra* is the most enjoyable. *Yoganidra* or yogic sleep brings about a state , where one is neither asleep nor fully awake. One drifts in and out of consciousness in the most pleasurable manner. Scientific experiments have shown that during this practice, the activities of the brain and heart slow down and the oxygen consumption is greatly reduced, indicating less work for the body tissues. The rest gives the tissues a chance to strengthen themselves perfectly. Even a short *Yoganidra* makes the practitioner feel fresh and rejuvenated. Though this technique can be practised anywhere in any position, doing it at the end of the day in Shavasana is the most effective. It releases the tension accumulated during the day and induces sound sleep which further rejuvenates the tissues. But it should not be practised immediately after a meal. Wait for two to three hours or till the stomach feels empty. *Yoganidra* should be practised in semi darkness for the best effect.

Technique

- Lie down in Shavasana.

- Visualize the body from top to toe.

- Consciously release the tension one by one from each part of the body where we generally hold it – forehead, eyebrows, eyelids, jaw, mouth, shoulders, chest, stomach, hips, right hand, left hand, right calf and left calf.

- Ensure that there is no tension anywhere in the body by again moving your mind over the said parts.

- Concentrate on your breath.

- Breathing should be absolutely normal.

- After 2-3 minutes, start counting the breaths backward from 27.

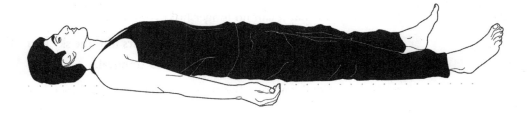

- Count 27 to 1 four times.
- Quickly move your mind over the following body parts.
- Right big toe, second toe, third toe, fourth, fifth, sole, heel, ankle, calf, knee, thigh, hip, waist, right shoulder, arm elbow, forearm, wrist, thumb, index finger, middle finger, ring finger and little finger.
- Repeat with the left side.
- Then — back, back of the neck, back of the head, top of the head, forehead, right eyebrow, left eyebrow, right eye, left eye, right cheek, left cheek, right ear, left ear, upper lip, lower lip, chin, chest, stomach and abdomen.
- The whole body is completely relaxed.
- Imagine your body is becoming lighter and lighter and still lighter.
- It is so light that it can no longer hold your soul in it.
- Your consciousness leaves the body and soars into the sky and to the space. The space is so peaceful, so tranquil.
- You are moving among the stars feeling so light and nice.

- Now you come back.

- You can see the earth as a tiny speck. It becomes bigger and bigger as you come closer.

- You come to the room where you had left your body.

- In the place of your body are seven lotus flowers arranged in a row.

- The lowest one is red with four petals, the next one has six petals which are crimson, the third is yellow with ten petals, the fourth has twelve blue petals, the fifth, a violet one, has sixteen petals and the second from the top has just two silver petals and the last one is a shiny lotus with a thousand petals.

- As you look at the flowers, admiring their beauty, a brilliant golden body of energy slowly appears around them. It solidifies, and it is *You*—but a much fresher and healthier you with a golden glow.

- Thanking the Almighty, you enter your body. Feel your body, move it a little and end the practice.

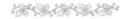

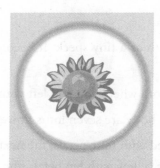

Tissue
Repairer

CHAPTER XI

Beauty is not possible without proper nutrition. Each of the nearly sixty trillion cells that constitute a human body need specific nutrients to remain whole and healthy. Any deficiency can easily damage them.

Another major source of damage to cells are the free radicals. These are molecules freed during oxidation process or are formed by factors such as radiation, pollutants and cigarette smoke. They are highly charged and electronically unbalanced. Unlike normal molecules these atoms do not have electrons in pairs. To rectify their inadequacy they try to get hold of electrons from other molecules, creating some other free radicals. Recocheting wildly, all these free radicals scar the tissues and distort their DNA. Viruses too cause extensive damage to the body cells by puncturing holes in them. As the tissues reproduce their exact replicas, these damaged tissues can only give rise to more faulty tissues and thus the degeneration sets in, picking up speed as time passes.

Therefore, the first step towards youth and beauty preservation, is an appropriate diet consisting of all the vitamins, minerals, fats, proteins, carbohydrates and that too in correct measure. It also should include anti-oxidants and

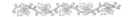

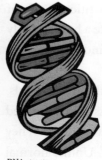

DNA structure

food rich in nucleic acids. Anti-oxidants counter the effects of free radicals and nucleic acids are the chief constituents of DNA and RNA.

Some *vaidyas* speak very highly of gold as an anti-ageing agent. Gold perhaps is the only metal that resists the harmful effects of oxygen. Oxygen, the life-giving element, unfortunately, destroys everything it comes in contact with. Iron rusts, silver tarnishes and so does copper. Gradually they are eroded. But nothing happens to gold. It remains the same. The presence of gold in the system is said to protect the tissues from the scarring effect of oxygen.

In Ayurveda, gold is considered to be heat producing, and so certain procedures are recommended for its ingestion to maintain the same body temperature. It is taken only during the peak of winter i.e. from mid-December to end-January; and it is generally taken with some cooling food such as *kheer* (a milk and rice preparation). Some even advise taking the *kheer* from a silver bowl as silver enhances the cooling. The purity of gold must be ensured. It should be nothing less than twenty-four carat. It can be taken as gold-leaf over eatables or better still as ash.

Some other wonder foods are:

Amla	a powerful anti-oxidant.
Almond	ensures smooth physiological functions.
Apple	removes toxic metals like lead and mercury from the blood; binds radioactive particles and eliminates them from the system.
Banana	apart from being an anti-oxidant, it prevents absorption of toxins by covering the naked surface of the digestive tract.
Chicken soup	repairs worn-out tissues.
Chilli	prevents absorption of toxins from the blood into the tissue.
Cabbage	promotes healthy collagen leading to a resilient and elastic skin.
Coconut	inactivates viruses.
Crab	retards ageing by keeping the nerves in perfect condition.
Fish	very rich in nucleic acids.
Garlic	diminishes oxidation.

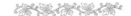

Grapes	anti-oxidant.
Green coconut	contains all important minerals.
Green gram	high in nucleic acids.
Jaggery (Gur)	cleans the system of pollutants.
Honey	maintains a sterile condition in the intestine.
Mint	removes chemicals from the blood.
Mushroom	a rich source of nucleic acid.
Onion	has a lethal effect on various germs and bacteria.
Potato	anti-oxidant
Toddy	increases nucleic acid in the system.
Turmeric	prevents DNA damage and also initiates its repair.
Wheat grass juice	an extremely powerful anti-oxidant.

For long people have been commenting how most Oriyas generally look much younger than their age. A little personal research revealed that it is the Oriya cuisine which is highly anti-ageing. Their food combinations and the mode of preparation are extremely health promoting and youth preserving.

Their staple diet is rice—mostly fermented; lots of green vegetables, especially the leafy variety; and fish, including crab. Fermented rice prevents liver damage and is full of vitamin B-complex while green leafy vegetables are a rich source of iron and calcium and are also powerful anti-oxidants. Here are a few simple Oriya recipies for you to try.

1. **Pakhal** - Take a cup of cooked rice in a bowl and pour three cups of water in it. Mix well, cover and keep it overnight in a warm place (it can be kept longer to ferment more but not longer than 24 hours as then the alcohol content would be too high). Add salt according to taste. You can also add green chillies and onion cut into small pieces.

    Pakhal induces sleep and is cooling. It should not be eaten in winters. Pakhal is usually taken with pan-fried fish and some of the following accompaniments.

2. **Baked Potato** - Wash a potato well and bake it on the stove with its skin on. Remove from fire when it feels soft. Let it cool naturally, and then take out the charred skin. Add chopped onion and chillies, salt to taste and a little water. Cut in small pieces. Add half a teaspoon of raw mustard oil. Lemon juice

or baked tomato (prepared in the similar manner) can also be added.

2. **Baked Brinjal** - same procedure as baked potatoes.

3. **Baked Ladyfinger** - same procedure as baked potatoes.

4. **Saag** - Take one or more variety of leaves – spinach, chaulai, leaves of beet, cauliflower, bitter gourd, pumpkin, drumstick, parwal and radish. Wash and cut.

   Heat oil, add mustard seeds and crushed garlic. Add some chopped vegetables such as potato, brinjal, green banana (raw), fry a little. Add the leaves, salt and cover. Simmer till cooked.

5. **Dalma** - Cook together – one cup green gram (split); one cup mixed vegetables (banana, pumpkin, potato and brinjal). ¼ tsp turmeric. Salt to taste. Cook till soft.

   In 1 tbs oil, crackle ½ tsp mustard seeds and add to the dish. Dry roast 1 tsp cumin seed till it gives out a nice aroma. Powder it roughly and sprinkle over Dalma and have it with plain boiled rice or coconut rice.

6. **Coconut Rice** - Wash and drain one cup of basmati rice. Mix with it ½ cup of scraped coconut, one bay leaf, 1 tsp ghee, one

black cardamom (crushed), ½ tsp pepper corn. 1 tbs aniseed powder, 1 tsp sugar and salt to taste. Add two cups of water— a little more is sometimes required. Pressure cook it till done.

7. **Fish Vegetables** - Cook one cup of cubed potatoes and one cup of cubed green bananas in one cup of water with ¼ tsp turmeric, 2 tsp mustard paste and salt to taste. Keeep aside.

   In 1 tbs oil, fry ½ onion till transluscent. Add two pieces of any salt water fish and fry till done. Remove from fire, cool and remove all bones.

   Heat 1 tbs oil in a pan. Put *paanchforan* (five spices)— *jeera* (cumin seed), *saunf* (aniseed), *kalaunji* (caraway seed), *methi* (fenugreek seed) and mustard. When they crackle, add ginger, garlic and *jeera* paste (1 tsp of each) and fry a little.

   Add cooked vegetables, fish and ¼ tsp cinnamon powder. Mix well and remove after five minutes.

   Temper with mustard seeds fried in cow's ghee.

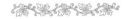

The

Illuminator

Ultimately, beauty comes from within—so goes the saying. Cliched—but true! A beautiful mind shines forth illuminating and transforming the most common face into an exceedingly charming one; whereas the beauty of an otherwise perfect face may not be so attractive if the person is dark from within.

Emotions manifest themselves through facial expressions. As time passes, these expressions leave permanent traces, more so when the skin starts losing its resilience with advancing age. Negative emotions such as anger, greed and jealousy leave their indelible marks on the face, robbing the softness of the features and distorting them for life.

Negative emotions also affect one's aura adversely, which can ruin relationships and bring unhappiness to the person — another factor that damages health and beauty. Each person is surrounded by an aura which reflects his or her physical and mental condition. Though the aura is invisible to the naked eye, the all-seeing, all-knowing subconscious sees it and recognises its qualities. We accept or reject a person on the basis of this subconscious reaction. Inexplicably we avoid a negative person while thousands get drawn to a saintly one. Various factors are responsible in creating negative emotions in a person.

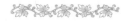

On the physical level, weak malfunctioning glands or organs can give rise to unwanted emotions. For example, overactive adrenal glands make a person short-tempered while under-active thyroid can lead to depression. Jaundiced view is a well-known phrase that describes a person with a sour attitude. A weak liver here is the culprit. Even certain diet deficiencies result in depression and irritation.

Hatha Yoga holds unbalanced energy responsible for an unbalanced personality. According to it, there are two types of energies flowing in the human body — physical and mental. They must remain at par with each other for a person to behave reasonably. If the physical energy is too much in excess of the mental energy, the person becomes aggressive, destructive and violent, often with criminal tendencies while the opposite can make the person introvert, neurotic or even insane.

A scarred psyche too leads to behavioural problems. Childhood trauma and the mother's thoughts while the baby is in her womb are held responsible for an abnormal psyche.

The last and the most deep-rooted factor comes from the spiritual level. According to yoga, the inner nature of a person depends on his or her stage of evolution. A person cannot but act and react according to his spiritual level. The soul is said to evolve from *chakra* to *chakra. Mooladhara Chakra* is the lowest *chakra* for humans and the highest one for animals. A *mooladhara* man, having just emerged out of the animal ancestery retains most of the animal qualities. Like animals, they live to survive. Food, shelter and procreation are their only concerns. They can turn violent – fighting physically, or even killing – in order to acquire or protect their basic needs. A person whose consciousness is at the next *chakra, Swadhisthana*, is less animal-like. But the person is still crude and loud. He is drawn to external show and glitter. For him, sensual pleasures are the most important factors. Devoid of any ethics or morals, he sets out to acquire wealth by any means which would enable him to satisfy his hunger.

The *Manipura* man leaves behind the crudity and thought-lessness of his earlier level. He is now more human; he thinks and reflects on the finer aspects of life. Though he still chases wealth, it is more for fame, status and power than to gratify his senses. Yearning to know one's true nature and the Divine, slowly manifests in the person after he leaves *Manipura*. The more he advances towards *Anahata* – the *chakra* near the heart, the more sensitive and refined he becomes. He feels and cares for others and sympathises genuinely with the downtrodden. And when he reaches *Anahata*, he is filled

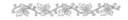

with love and compassion. He ceases to think for himself, devoting all his time to improve others' lives. He becomes a saint, propagating the message of peace and universal love.

Beyond *Anahata* lies the domain of the Divine. As the individual soul advances in this area he manifests divine qualities more and more. In *Agnya* – the *chakra* of the third eye, he knows everything – past, present and future. He can read other's thoughts and he heals with just a word, touch or a thought. By the time he reaches *Sahasrara* – the highest *chakra* – he is no less a God himself. His consciousness is merged with that of the Supreme.

No matter what the reason is for a person's negative emotions, yoga can change that. To rectify the glandular problems and to balance the subtle energies, Hatha Yoga practices are excellent while meditation works wonder with the mind and psyche. Many criminals who are made to practise meditation completely give up their criminal tendencies.

But ultimately meditation is a spiritual practice that takes you to higher planes. Faith, prayer, ritualistic worship, singing *bhajan* and *kirtan*, listening to religious and spiritual discourses, self-enquiry, intense love for the downtrodden, unconditional devotion to one's guru and selfless service are also means to evolve.

There are any number of meditative techniques in the world, each being as good as the other. But one must choose a technique that suits one's temperament and condition. Only then can one practise it with sincerity. The great saint Swami Sivananda of Rishikesh recommends meditation on virtues to change the inner nature.

And thus yoga and meditation normalise physiological functions, soothe and strengthen frayed nerves; calm the mind; clear the psyche of all negative elements and make us evolve to become better human beings.

To Tone Up the Nervous System

TRIKON (SEE CHAPTER II)

EK PADA PRANAMASANA

Technique

- Stand straight.
- Place the right sole on the left thigh just above the knee.
- Fold hands near the chest.
- Look straight ahead and breathe normally.

- Hold the posture steadily for 20 breaths.
- Change legs and repeat.

To Strengthen the Glandular System (See Chapter V)

To Counter Anger

SHASHANKASANA (NORMALISES ADRENAL FUNCTION)

Technique
- Sit in Vajrasana.
- Inhaling, raise hands above.
- Exhaling, bend forward and place your forehead and forearms on the floor.
- Breathe normally.

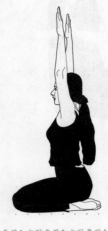

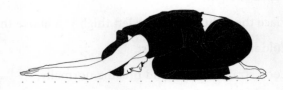

- Remain in this posture for five minutes to half-an-hour, depending on the intensity of the problem.

To Calm Down Quickly

OUM CHANTING

- Sit in any position.
- Take a deep breath.
- Exhale deeply through the mouth while saying O…….U…….M…….aloud.
- Try to maintain a uniform pitch.
- Repeat 7, 13 or 27 times depending on the time available.

OUM REPETITION

- Mentally say 'O' while you inhale and 'um' when you exhale.
- The breathing should be spontaneous.
- Alternatively repeat it faster – one Oum per second.

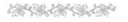

- These techniques can be followed any time, anywhere and in any position to release stress quickly.

MEDITATION ON VIRTUES

Decide the virtue you want to cultivate. Remember the word. Do not change it till you succeed.

- Sit down in a meditative pose.

- Close your eyes.

- Consciously release the tension from various body parts such as the forehead, eyebrows, eyelids, jaw, mouth, shoulder, right hand, left hand, chest, stomach, hips, right thigh, left thigh, right calf and left calf.

- Inhale slowly and deeply.

- Exhale deeply.

- Repeat seven times.

- Breathe normally and concentrate on it. If the mind wanders follow it for a while then bring it back to your breath.

- Continue for five minutes or so.

- Mentally repeat the chosen word like a *mantra*... peace, peace, peace... for 2-3 minutes.

- Visualise the peaceful faces of great saints, gurus and prophets, one by one – contemplating one person for some time.

- Imagine peace emanating from them, engulfing you, soaking to the very depth of your being.

- Feel truly peaceful.

- Visualise yourself dealing with an adverse situation without losing your composure.

- Say to yourself mentally – *I am so peaceful.*

- Repeat the sentence a few times more.

- Feel nice about your success and smile to yourself.

- Be aware of your surroundings.

- Open your eyes.

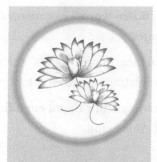

Mantras
and
Tidbits

CHAPTER XIII

Our physical body is subjected to harsh treatment by the sun, wind, water and pollutants. These elements affect it adversely making it dry and dirty. Therefore, external care should be combined with internal care to protect the body from nature's fury. Ignoring it can only diminish the effects of our efforts to remain young and healthy. In the external treatment, the skin takes the priority.

Apart from being the largest beauty feature, the skin also acts as agent to flush out pollutants. The body discards a lot of toxins through the pores of the skin. For the skin to function properly, the pores need to be kept clean. If the pores are clogged, it cannot discard toxins adequately and the toxicity of blood increases, giving rise to many problems including that of the skin. It also increases the load on the other body organs, namely the liver and the kidneys. These get tired and can't do their job properly. Thus a chain reaction is set in the system, making it dirtier and unhealthier by the day.

Traditionally, mud or gram flour was used to cleanse the skin. Apart from cleansing it deeply, they also nourish the skin. Soil is full of life giving *prana* and many minerals, while gram is a rich source of proteins and vitamins. Once in a while it should be used to clean the body. Turmeric (*haldi*) application is another tradition and practice which is extremely beneficial to repair DNA that gets damaged by the sun. It should be applied all over the body at least once a week and kept for an hour before washing it. In many homes, turmeric is applied a day in advance and left overnight prior to religious ceremonies. It can then be washed off with mud or gram flour. If necessary, soap can be used later.

Nourishing the skin replaces vital nutrients lost to the environment. Milk, the complete food, feeds the skin well. Facial skin is the worst affected and needs still more nourishment. Honey, almond and fruits are excellent facial tonics. They can be mixed together and applied or can be used separately. Honey is a natural bleach too.

Skin should be exfoliated before applying the nourishments. Otherwise, the uppermost layer of the skin, which is nothing but dead cells, prevent the food from going to the active inner cells. Also, when dead cells are removed, new cells are exposed, making the skin look young and fresh.

The skin should also receive adequate blood supply to remain healthy. The amount of blood flow to skin diminishes if the thin blood capillaries are not relaxed. Yogic relaxation techniques such as *Yoganidra* relaxes the blood capillaries and rectifies this problem. Body massage is also effective to improve blood flow to the skin.

Ayurveda has an interesting method for skin rejuvenation. It is called *Kayakalpa*. The treatment lasts over a month and during that period the person is required to remain underground. The skin is peeled off bit by bit using natural abrasives like raw garlic paste. A smooth baby skin is thus encouraged to form. *Kayakalpa* is a precise and complicated process which is best handled by experienced *vaidyas*.

EYE CARE

Eyes are our most precious possession. We interact with people through our eyes. At the same time the beauty aspect of eyes cannot be denied. Clean sparkling eyes are a visual delight while blood red, tired ones are a beauty detractor. Rest and exercise are the most important things for optic health – so is keeping them cool and clean.

In yoga, *netra dhauti* is advised to keep the eyes clean and *tratak* is practised to maintain eye-sight. Vedic life calls for a ritual that involves reciting a *stotra* while holding some water in the hands . To rest the eyes every now and then one should practise a yogic technique called palming.

Ayurveda recommends *amla* (Indian Gooseberry) wash and rose water drops to guard eye health. Practise as many of these methods as you can.

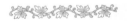

Netra Dhauti

- Fill your mouth with water. Splash water 20 to 40 times into the eyes.

- Practise it in the morning after you have brushed your teeth.

Amla Wash

- Soak a piece of dry amla in a cup of water. Strain and wash your eyes with it. You can use a eye glass for convenience.

Rose Water

- This is done to brighten up the eyes. Put a drop of pure rose water into each eye. If it is concentrated, dilute it with cold water. Pads soaked in rose water can also be kept over the closed eyes while you lie down and relax. This too has a soothing effect on eyes.

Tratak

- Place a candle in front of you at eye level and at a distance of one arm's length

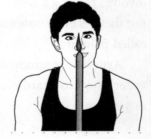

- Stare at its brightest spot without blinking, till your eyes water, or for one to two minutes.

- Close eyes. You will be able to see the after image of the flame quite clearly. Try to hold it in between your eyebrows and focus on it. When the image fades, open the eyes.

- Repeat it three times.

- After a month or so, some other object such as a black dot or a flower should be used instead of the candle.

Palming

- Rub your hands till they are warm.

- Lightly place them on the closed eyelids and feel the warmth flooding the eyes.

- After a few seconds remove hands.

- Repeat 5-10 times.

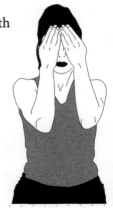

STOTRA (A GROUP OF MANTRAS MAKE A STOTRA)

*Om Asyashchakschushividyaya Ahiburdhnya Rishirgayatri
Chhandah Suryo Devata Chakschuroganivrttaye Viniyogah.*

*Om Chakschu Chakschu Chakschu Tejah Sthiro Bhava
Mam Pahi Pahi*

Twaritam Chakschurogan Shamaya Shamaya

Mama Jatarupam Tejo Darshaya Darshaya

Yatha Aham Andho Na Syam Tatha Kalpaya Kalpaya

Kalyanam Kuru Kuru

*Yani Mama Purvajanmoparjitani Chakschu
Pratirodhakadushkritani Sarvani Nirmulaya Nirmulaya*

Om Namah Chakschustejodatre Divyaya Bhaskaraya

Om Namah Karunakarayamritaya

Om Namah Suryaya

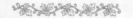

Om Namo Bhagvate Suryayakshitejase Namah

Khechraya Namah

Mahate Namah

Rajase Namah

Tamase Namah

Asato Ma Sadgamaya

Tamaso Ma Jyotirgamaya

Mrityorma Amritam Gamaya

Ushno Bhagvanchhuchirupah

Hanso Bhagwan Shuchirpratirupah

Facing the morning sun with water in the palms, recite the stotra and then pour the water out as offering it to the sun.

KAJAL

The use of Kajal too is highly recommended by Ayurveda. Cow's *ghee* that is used in *kajal* is supposed to ward off infections. To ensure the purity of *kajal*, it should be made at home.

The soot from a castor oil lamp can be collected by covering the flame with an inverted iron bowl or spoon. It should then be mixed with just enough cow's *ghee* to form a tight lump.

HAIR CARE

Hair, like skin, should be washed, nourished and massaged regularly. *Ritha, shikkakai* and mud are the best natural cleansing agents while coconut oil provides the necessary nourishment.

Red hibiscus flower, according to Ayurveda, is good to nourish hair. The Mother Goddess with her luxuriant flowing hair is worshipped only with this flower. One wonders if it is an indication that hibiscus is meant for hair growth. Hibiscus can be rubbed into the scalp or put into the hair oil for convenience. Generally twenty flowers are put in half a kilo of pure coconut oil and kept in the sun for one month before use. Strain and remove the flowers. One tablespoon of fenugreek seeds can also be added to it to prevent dandruff.

To cure dandruff problem, application of old sour curd together with fenugreek powder on the scalp is extremely effective.

Combing hair with a hard horn comb especially of buffalo's horn strengthens the roots. It should be done in Vajrasana while repeating the mantra *sheeth* for best result. Do it for ten minutes after meals.

To darken grey hair naturally, amla powder mixed with mango kernel powder can be used. Only raw mangoes can be used (before their kernels have hardened). These should be sun dried and preserved for the whole year. Though it does not hide the whiteness completely, and bleeds colour when washed, many prefer it to chemical dyes.

The following *asana* brings a rich supply of blood to the hair roots and improves their health.

Pranamasana

Technique

- Sit in Vajrasana.
- Hold your calves.
- Take a deep breath.

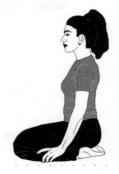
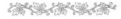

- Exhaling, bend forward and keep the head on the floor.
- Retaining the breath inside, lift the hips up while rolling the head to let the corner of the head take the weight.
- Hold the posture for some time.
- Lower the hips while rolling back the head.
- Inhaling, lift the head and return to the upright sitting position.
- Repeat five times.

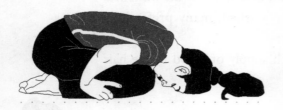 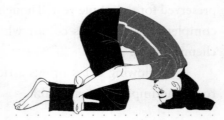

ORAL CARE

Teeth should be cleaned with a *datun* (twig) for good health, neem being the best choice. It kills germs in the mouth and prevents caries and gum diseases. The *datun* is chewed on one end to make it into a brush.

The chewing hardens the gums. A twig from the guava tree is a good substitute. It can be dipped in honey and used as a brush. Honey is an antiseptic and a natural bleach.

After meals a few grains of salt should be put in the mouth to dislodge food particles and to kill germs. There is a saying which goes *Ante tikta, dante non, pet bharon ko hai teen kon* – which means, bitter should be in the intestine and salt in the teeth and only three quarter of the stomach should be filled.

Ayurveda recommends oil gargle for better oral health. It is done in the morning with seasme seed (*til*) oil, using only the frontal part and not involving the throat. It is also said to maintain a firm jawline and an unlined face.

LIP CARE

A drop of oil, preferably mustard, put into the navel prevents chapping of the lips.

FASTING

The pituitary gland secretes growth hormone which is crucial for growth as well as the repair of body cells. The secretion is found to be better during fasting and non-aerobic exercises like yoga. Hence, keep a fast once a week but for not more than twenty-four hours.

SELF TALKING

The cells of our body have the intelligence to understand our wishes and act accordingly. When we want to blink our eyes, the cells of our eyelids close and open. When we want to walk, the cells of our legs carry us forward. So on and so forth. Normally it is the brain which receives our wishes and passes on the command to the relevant body part. But we can also make them work by passing a direct order. I have tried this technique on many of my students with wonderful results.

(Should be practised immediately after meditation or *Yoganidra*)

Technique

- Visualise the body part you want to speak to.

- Imagine it having a face with eyes, nose and lips.

- Speak to it normally but firmly.

- Visualise it say '*Yes sir, your wish is my command*'.

- Visualise it carrying out your order exactly the way you want it.

- Smile lovingly at it.

- Visualise it smiling back.

- Pat it in appreciation.

- You can actually pat it if you so wish.

- Feel nice and healthy. Open your eyes.

Guide

All yogic techniques are excellent, but it is not possible to practise all of them every day. Here is a guide to help you progress in the most practical way.

1. Normalise your blood pressure.

    (*Most of the yogic techniques mentioned in this book are not for people with heart problems, hernia, severe back problems etc. In case of other ailments, consult a medical practitioner before practising yoga from books.*)

2. Rectify mild spinal ailments if you have any. All forward bending asanas, except Shashankasana, worsen back ailments (for details, see author's book *Yoga to Banish Backache*).

3. Write down all your problems and the recommended yogic practices.

4. If you are a beginner, follow the one-week programme first from the book *Yoga for Busy People*, to attune your body to yoga.

5. Shed all the extra weight by appropriate *asanas* and diet.

6. If possible, practise *Guru Shankh Prakshyalan* first under an expert. After this practice, the effect of yoga is enhanced manifold.

7. Divide your yogic routine into two or three segments

   I. Slimming

   II. Toning and general fitness, and

   III. Anti-ageing.

   Practise each segment twice a week, say Monday and Thursday for one segment; Tuesday and Friday for the second one, and Wednesday and Saturday for the third.

   Important - *Bandhas* should be attempted only after a year of yoga practice.

8. Keep weekends for cleansing, massage and turmeric application. Hair oil can be applied the night before.

9. One must meditate every day and at the same time. So choose a time when you are normally free.

10. Do not let stress remain in the system. Practise *Yoganidra* or

Oum repetition whenever you are tense.

11. At night, reflect on your actions of the day and resolve to rectify the shortcomings.

12. Practise *Guru Shankha Prakshyalana* whenever you get a chance—but not more than once a year.

13. Last, but not the least, be a little careful with what you do. It makes no sense to practise yoga to attain and maintain good health and lose it all by following a damaging lifestyle. So do whatever you fancy — eat and drink whatever you like, go out or party — but all in moderation. It will certainly pay off in the long run.

Reference

1. *Nutrients A to Z*, Dr. Michael Sharon, Rupa & Co.

2. *Medicinal Secrets of Your Food*, Dr. Aman

3. *I am Joe's Body*, J. D. Ritcliff, Berkley Books, New York

4. *Mayo Clinic Family Health Book*, Published by William Morrow & Company, Inc., New York

5. *Health and Hygiene*, Swami Sivananda, Divine Life Society

6. *Mind – Its Mysteries and Control*, Swami Sivananda, Divine Life Society

7. *Autobiography of a Yogi*, Paramahamsa Yogananda

8. *Hatha Yoga Pradipika*, Bihar School of Yoga, Munger

9. *Asana Pranayama Mudra Bandha*, Swami Satyananda Saraswati, Bihar School of Yoga, Munger

10. *Ramma Bans Book of Health and Beauty*, Ramma Bans

11. *The Science of Psychic Healing*, Yogi Ramacharaka

Index